RISING ABOVE CANCER

A Story of Strength, Courage, and Hope

BY
Dr. JOANNA WELLS

Book review

Rising Above Cancer is an inspiring and informative book that offers hope, encouragement, and practical advice to those who have been diagnosed with cancer. Written by **Dr. Joanna Wells**, a cancer survivor, the book explores the author's journey through diagnosis, treatment, and recovery. It also provides readers with insights into how to navigate the many challenges that come with a cancer diagnosis.

The book covers a range of topics, including coping with the emotional impact of a cancer diagnosis, making informed decisions about treatment options, managing the side effects of treatment, and maintaining a healthy lifestyle during and after treatment. The author's personal experiences are woven throughout the book, making it a relatable and engaging read.

Overall, **Rising Above Cancer** is a valuable resource for anyone who has been affected by cancer. It provides practical advice and encouragement to help readers navigate the complex journey of cancer treatment and recovery.

Copyright

The information and advice contained in **Rising Above Cancer** by **Dr. Joanna Wells** are intended to provide helpful and informative material on the subject of cancer and its treatments. Nonetheless, the information provided is not intended to replace or substitute professional medical advice, diagnosis, or treatment.

The author and publisher of this book disclaim any liability or responsibility for any direct, indirect, or consequential loss or damage resulting from the use of the information contained in this book.

Readers should always seek the advice of a qualified healthcare provider with any questions they may have regarding their health or a medical condition. They should not disregard professional medical advice or delay in seeking it because of something they have read in this book or any other source

Table of content

1.
2.
3.

1.

1.
2.

1.
2.
3.
4.
5.

1.
2.

1.
2.
3.
4.

Introduction

The journey ahead

Cancer is a disease that involves the uncontrolled growth and spread of abnormal cells in the body. The journey ahead of cancer depends on various factors, including the type and stage of cancer, the treatment options available, and the patient's overall health.

Here is a general overview of the journey ahead for cancer:

1. Diagnosis: The journey begins with a diagnosis, which may involve a physical exam, medical history, and diagnostic tests such as imaging tests, blood tests, or biopsies.
2. Staging: Once cancer is diagnosed, the next step is to determine the stage of cancer. Staging helps doctors determine the extent of cancer, including whether it has spread to other parts of the body.
3. Treatment planning: Based on the cancer type and stage, doctors will develop a treatment plan that may

involve one or more treatments, including surgery, radiation therapy, chemotherapy, targeted therapy, immunotherapy, or a combination of these.

4. Treatment: The actual treatment process can be challenging and may include hospital stays, outpatient appointments, and multiple rounds of treatment.

5. Monitoring and follow-up: After treatment, patients will need to be closely monitored to ensure that the cancer does not return. Follow-up care may include regular check-ups, imaging tests, and blood tests.

6. Survivorship: For some patients, cancer treatment can be successful, and they will seeenter survivorship. This phase involves ongoing monitoring, managing potential side effects of treatment, and making lifestyle changes to reduce the risk of cancer recurrence.

7. End-of-life care:
Unfortunately, some
patients may reach a point
where cancer treatment is
no longer effective. End-
of-life care involves
providing comfort and
support to patients and
their families during the
final stages of cancer.
8. Overall, the journey ahead
of cancer can be
challenging and emotional,
but with proper treatment
and care, many patients
can successfully manage
their cancer and enter
survivorship.

Chapter 1

Understanding cancer

A. Causes of cancer

Cancer is a polygenic disease
that can be caused by various
factors. Here are some of the
known causes of cancer:

1. Genetic mutations:
Changes in the DNA
sequence can cause normal
cells to become cancerous.

These mutations can be inherited or acquired over time due to exposure to carcinogens.

2. Carcinogens: Certain substances or agents in the environment can cause genetic mutations that can lead to cancer. Examples of carcinogens include tobacco smoke, radiation, and certain chemicals.

3. Viruses: Some viruses, such as human papillomavirus (HPV), hepatitis B and C viruses (HBV and HCV), and human immunodeficiency virus (HIV), can cause cancer by disrupting the normal function of cells.

4. Lifestyle factors: Poor diet, lack of physical activity, obesity, and excessive alcohol consumption can increase the risk of developing certain types of cancer.

5. Age: The risk of developing cancer increases as people age, as the accumulation of genetic mutations over

time increases the likelihood of cancerous cell growth.

6. Hormones: Hormones such as estrogen and testosterone can play a role in the development of certain cancers, such as breast and prostate cancer.
7. Family history: Some types of cancer, such as breast, ovarian, and colon cancer, can run in families due to inherited genetic mutations.

It's important to note that not all cancers have a clear cause and that many cancers are likely caused by a combination of factors. Additionally, having one or more risk factors does not necessarily mean a person will develop cancer, as many people with risk factors never develop the disease.

B. Symptoms of cancer

The manifestations of cancer can differ based on the kind and progression of the disease. Some common symptoms may include:

1. Fatigue or weakness
2. Unexplained weight loss

3. Pain or discomfort, especially if it persists
4. Changes in the skin, such as darkening or yellowing, or the appearance of new moles or growths
5. A persistent cough or hoarseness
6. Difficulty swallowing or persistent indigestion
7. Changes in bowel or bladder habits, such as diarrhea or constipation, blood in urine or stool, or frequent urination
8. Unexplained fever or night sweats
9. Swelling or lumps in the neck, underarm, stomach, or groin
10. Abnormal bleeding or discharge, such as from the vagina, nipples, or rectum.

It is important to note that having one or more of these symptoms does not necessarily mean that you have cancer, but it is important to consult a healthcare professional if you are facing any continous or concerning symptoms. Early detection and

treatment are crucial for
successful cancer management.

C. Diagnostics of cancer

The diagnosis of cancer typically
involves several steps, including:

1. Medical history and
   physical examination: The
   doctor will ask about your
   symptoms, medical
   history, and family history
   of cancer. They will also
   perform a physical
   examination to check for
   any lumps, bumps, or
   other abnormalities.
2. Imaging tests: Imaging
   tests, such as X-rays, CT
   scans, MRI scans, and
   ultrasounds, can be used to
   detect tumors and
   determine their size and
   location.
3. Biopsy: A biopsy is a
   procedure in which a small
   piece of tissue is removed
   from the suspected tumor
   and examined under a
   microscope. This is the
   conclusive way to
   diagnose cancer.
4. Blood tests: Blood tests
   can be used to check for

certain markers that may
indicate the presence of
cancer.

Once a diagnosis of cancer is made, additional tests may be done to determine the stage of cancer and to help guide treatment decisions. These may include:

1. Staging tests: Staging tests, such as bone scans, PET scans, and CT scans, can help determine the extent of cancer and whether it has spread to other parts of the body.

2. Molecular testing: Molecular testing can help identify specific genetic mutations or biomarkers that may be targeted by certain cancer treatments.

The specific diagnostic tests used will depend on the type and location of the suspected cancer, as well as the individual patient's medical history and other factors. It's important to work closely with your healthcare team to determine the most appropriate diagnostic tests for your situation.

Chapter 2

Navigating the Healthcare System:

A. Finding the right doctors and support services

This process can be a daunting task, but it is an important step in managing your illness and improving your quality of life. Here are some tips to help you find the right doctors and support services:

1. Talk to your primary care physician: Your primary care physician can be a valuable resource for finding the right doctors and support services. They can refer you to specialists and provide you with information on support services in your area.

2. Research online: There are many online resources available to help you find doctors and support services. You can use search engines like Google

or visit websites like the American Cancer Society to find information on doctors and support services.

3. Check with your insurance company: Your insurance company can provide you with a list of doctors and support services that are covered under your plan. This can help you narrow down your options and make an informed decision.

4. Ask for recommendations: You can ask friends, family, or support groups for recommendations on doctors and support services. They may have had experience with certain providers and can provide valuable insights.

5. Consider location and convenience: When selecting doctors and support services, consider their location and convenience. You may want to choose providers who are close to your home or work to make it

easier for you to attend appointments.

6. Ask questions: When you meet with doctors and support services, don't be afraid to ask questions. Ask about their experience with cancer patients, their treatment philosophy, and their approach to patient care.

7. Trust your instincts: Ultimately, you should trust your instincts when selecting doctors and support services. If something doesn't feel right, or you don't feel comfortable with a provider, it's okay to seek out other options.

Remember, finding the right doctors and support services is an important step in managing your cancer diagnosis. Don't be afraid to take the time to research and ask questions to find the best providers for your needs.

Chapter 3

Nutrition and exercise

A. Healthy Eating During Cancer

Eating well during cancer treatment is important for maintaining strength and energy, managing treatment side effects, and supporting overall health. Here are some tips for eating well during cancer:

1. Focus on nutrient-dense foods: Eat foods that are rich in nutrients such as fruits, vegetables, whole grains, lean protein, and healthy fats.
2. Stay hydrated: Drink plenty of fluids to help prevent dehydration, which can make you feel tired and weak. Aim for at least 8 glasses of water a day.
3. Manage treatment side effects: Some cancer treatments can cause side effects like nausea, vomiting, and mouth sores. Speak to your healthcare team to find out

what foods and drinks can
help manage these side
effects.

4. Eat small, frequent meals:
    Eating small, frequent
    meals throughout the day
    can help you maintain
    your energy levels and
    prevent nausea.

5. Consider nutritional
    supplements: If you're
    having trouble meeting
    your nutritional needs
    through food alone, your
    healthcare team may
    recommend nutritional
    supplements to help you
    get the nutrients you need.

6. Limit processed and
    sugary foods: Foods that
    are high in sugar and
    processed foods can be
    low in nutrients and may
    not provide the energy you
    need.

7. Stay active: Exercise and
    physical activity can help
    improve your energy
    levels, reduce stress, and
    improve your overall
    health.

It's important to speak to your
healthcare team to develop a

personalized nutrition plan that takes into account your individual needs and treatment plan. They can help you manage any side effects and make sure you're getting the nutrients you need to stay strong and healthy during your cancer treatment.

Exercise during cancer

The role of exercise during cancer treatment can vary depending on the type of cancer, the stage of cancer, and the overall health of the individual. However, in general, exercise is recommended during cancer treatment to help improve physical function, reduce fatigue, improve mood, and enhance overall quality of life. Below are written things to keep in mind:

1. Talk to your healthcare team: Before starting any exercise program, it is important to talk to your healthcare team to ensure it is safe for you to do so. They can provide you with guidance on any precautions or adaptations you may need to undertake

2. Start slow: If you have not been exercising regularly, start with low-intensity activities such as walking, yoga or swimming. Gradually increase the duration and intensity of your workouts as you feel comfortable.

3. Listen to your body: It is important to listen to your body and adjust your workout intensity or duration if you are experiencing fatigue or other symptoms related to cancer or cancer treatment.

4. Stay hydrated: It is important to stay hydrated during exercise, especially if you are undergoing chemotherapy or radiation therapy.

5. Get enough rest: Getting enough rest is crucial for your body to recover and heal. Avoid overdoing it and give yourself plenty of time to rest and recover between workouts.

6. Stay active: Even if you are not up for a full workout, try to stay active

by taking short walks or doing gentle stretches throughout the day. This can help prevent muscle weakness and maintain mobility.

Overall, exercise can be a valuable tool during cancer treatment. Consult with your healthcare team to develop an exercise program that is safe and appropriate for you.

Chapter 4

Managing symptoms

Pain Management:

Cancer can cause a great deal of physical and emotional pain, and effective pain management is an essential part of cancer treatment. Here are some approaches to pain management during cancer:

1. Medications: Pain medication is often prescribed to manage cancer pain. Depending on the type and severity of the pain, different types of medication may be used,

including opioids, nonsteroidal anti-inflammatory drugs (NSAIDs), and other drugs like anticonvulsants or antidepressants. These medications can be taken orally, through injection, or via skin patches.

2. Complementary therapies: Complementary therapies such as acupuncture, massage, meditation, and relaxation techniques can also be used to manage cancer pain. These therapies can help reduce anxiety and stress, which can worsen pain.

3. Supportive care: supportive care is a type of care that focuses on managing symptoms and improving quality of life. It can involve a team of healthcare providers, including doctors, nurses, and social workers, who work together to manage pain and other symptoms.

4. Radiation therapy: Radiation therapy can be used to shrink tumors that

are causing pain, which
can help relieve pain.

5. Surgery: In some cases, surgery may be necessary to remove tumors or other cancer-related issues that are causing pain.

It's essential to work closely with your healthcare team to determine the best pain management approach for you. Pain is subjective and can vary greatly from person to person, so what is effective in relieving pain for one individual may not be effective for another. Regular communication with your healthcare team is key to managing cancer pain effectively.

Fatigue Management:

Fatigue is a common symptom experienced by cancer patients, which can have a significant impact on their quality of life. Managing cancer-related fatigue involves a multi-disciplinary approach, which includes medical management, lifestyle modifications, and psychosocial support.

Here are some tips for managing fatigue during cancer:

1. Physical activity: Regular physical activity, such as walking, yoga, or swimming, can help improve fatigue levels. It is essential to speak with your healthcare provider before starting any exercise routine.

2. Sleep hygiene: Getting enough restful sleep is crucial for managing fatigue. Ensure a comfortable sleep environment, avoid daytime naps, and establish a consistent bedtime routine.

3. Balanced diet: Eating a balanced diet that includes a variety of fruits, vegetables, whole grains, lean proteins, and healthy fats can provide the body with the necessary nutrients for energy and vitality.

4. Medications: Sometimes, cancer treatments can cause fatigue. Your medical practitioner may

recommend medications as
part of your treatment plan
to alleviate your
symptoms.
5. Relaxation techniques:
Activities like meditation,
deep breathing, and
massage therapy can help
reduce stress, which can
contribute to fatigue.
6. Support system: Talking to
loved ones, joining a
support group, or seeing a
mental health professional
can provide emotional
support and help alleviate
fatigue symptoms.
7. Time management:
Prioritizing important
activities, taking breaks
when needed, and
delegating tasks to others
can help manage fatigue
and conserve energy.

It's essential to work with your
healthcare provider to determine
the best fatigue management plan
for you. Remember to be patient
and kind to yourself, as
managing cancer-related fatigue
can take time and effort.

Nausea and Vomiting

Nausea and vomiting are common symptoms experienced by cancer patients, particularly those undergoing chemotherapy or radiation therapy. There are various approaches that can be employed to effectively manage these symptoms.

1. Medications: Anti-nausea medications, also known as antiemetics, can be prescribed by your doctor to help manage nausea and vomiting. These medications may be given before or after chemotherapy or radiation therapy. There are several different types of antiemetics, including serotonin receptor antagonists, dopamine receptor antagonists, and corticosteroids.

2. Acupuncture: Acupuncture is an alternative therapy that has been shown to reduce nausea and vomiting in cancer patients. Acupuncture involves the precise

insertion of fine needles into specific points on the body to enhance the flow of energy.

3. Ginger: Ginger has anti-inflammatory properties that may help reduce nausea and vomiting. It can be taken in various forms, including as a tea or in capsule form.

4. Relaxation techniques: Relaxation techniques such as deep breathing, meditation, and guided imagery can help reduce stress and anxiety, which can contribute to nausea and vomiting.

5. Diet modification: Eating small, frequent meals and avoiding spicy or greasy foods may help reduce nausea and vomiting.It's crucial to maintain adequate hydration levels by consuming sufficient fluids.

It is important to talk to your doctor about your symptoms and any treatments you are considering. They can help you determine the best course of action for managing your nausea and vomiting.

Hair Loss

Hair loss is a common side effect of many cancer treatments, such as chemotherapy and radiation therapy. Managing hair loss during cancer can be challenging, but there are several strategies that can help.

1. Scalp cooling: Scalp cooling involves wearing a specialized cap during chemotherapy to lower the temperature of the scalp and reduce the amount of chemotherapy drugs that reach the hair follicles. This can reduce hair loss or make it less severe.
2. Wigs: Wearing a wig can help cover hair loss and boost self-confidence. Wigs can be made of synthetic or human hair, and there are many different styles and colors to choose from.
3. Scarves and hats: Scarves and hats are another option for covering hair loss. They are more

comfortable to wear than wigs, especially in warmer weather.

4. Hair care: During cancer treatment, it is important to be gentle with your hair. Use a mild shampoo and avoid using heat styling tools, such as hair dryers and curling irons. To prevent hair breakage, it is recommended to comb your hair with a wide-toothed comb instead of a brush.

5. Nutritional support: Eating a well-balanced diet that includes plenty of protein, vitamins, and minerals can help promote healthy hair growth. Consult with a registered dietitian for guidance.

6. Emotional support: Hair loss can be emotionally distressing. It is important to seek emotional support from friends, family, or a professional counselor to help cope with the changes to your appearance.

It is important to talk to your healthcare provider about any

concerns you have about hair
loss during cancer treatment.
They can offer extra assistance
and encouragement to help you.

Emotional Distress:

Receiving a cancer diagnosis can
be an overwhelming and
emotional experience. Coping
with the physical and emotional
aspects of cancer can be
challenging, but there are
strategies that can help manage
emotional distress during cancer.
Here are some tips:

1. Seek support: Talking to
   family, friends, and other
   loved ones about your
   feelings can be helpful.
   You can also join a
   support group for cancer
   patients or seek out a
   therapist or counselor who
   specializes in cancer-
   related issues.
2. Practice relaxation
   techniques: Relaxation
   techniques such as deep
   breathing, progressive
   muscle relaxation, and
   guided imagery can help
   reduce stress and anxiety.

3. Stay active: Exercise can help reduce stress, boost your mood, and improve your overall health. Even light activity like walking can make a big difference.

4. Engage in enjoyable activities: Doing things you enjoy can help distract you from your worries and boost your mood. Whether it's reading a book, watching a movie, or spending time with loved ones, make time for activities that make you happy.

5. Practice self-care: Taking care of yourself physically and emotionally can help you cope with the challenges of cancer. This includes eating a healthy diet, getting enough rest, and engaging in activities that promote self-care such as meditation or yoga.

6. Stay informed but avoid overwhelming information: It's important to stay informed about your cancer and treatment options, but too much

information can be overwhelming. Stick to trusted sources and limit your exposure to news and social media.

7. Talk to your healthcare team: Your healthcare team can provide support and resources to help manage emotional distress. Don't be afraid to ask questions or seek guidance from your doctor, nurse, or social worker.

Remember, it's normal to experience a range of emotions during cancer. Be kind to yourself and seek support when you need it.

Chapter 5

Life after cancer

Life after cancer refers to the period following a cancer diagnosis, where the individual has completed treatment and is transitioning back to their daily life. It can be a time of physical, emotional, and practical adjustments as the person tries to find a new normal.

Physically, the body may be weakened or altered from cancer treatment, and there may be lingering side effects. It's crucial to allow the body sufficient time to recuperate and restore itself. Engaging in regular physical activity and following a healthy diet can help improve overall health and wellness.

Emotionally, the experience of cancer can be traumatic and can take a toll on mental health. Many people experience anxiety, depression, or PTSD following a cancer diagnosis. Seeking support from a therapist, support group, or loved ones can help individuals process their emotions and cope with the changes in their life.

Practically, life after cancer may involve adjusting to changes in work, finances, or relationships. Individuals may need to make modifications to their work schedule or workload, adjust to changes in income or insurance coverage, or navigate changes in their relationships with friends and family.

Despite the challenges of life after cancer, many individuals find a renewed appreciation for life and a deeper sense of purpose. They may feel a sense of gratitude for each day and a desire to make the most of their time. Some individuals even find new passions or purpose through advocacy work, volunteering, or other activities that support the cancer community.

Ultimately, life after cancer is a journey unique to each individual. It's important to give oneself time and space to process the experience, seek support when needed, and focus on creating a fulfilling life beyond cancer.

The life of a cancer survivor after treatment can vary depending on many factors such as the type of cancer, the stage at which it was diagnosed, the treatment received, and the individual's overall health and wellbeing. However, some general aspects of life after cancer treatment may include:

1. Physical Changes: Treatment for cancer can cause physical changes in

the body, such as hair loss, weight changes, fatigue, and decreased physical functioning. Some of these changes may be temporary, while others may be permanent.

2. Emotional Impact: The emotional impact of cancer can be significant and long-lasting. Survivors may experience anxiety, depression, fear of recurrence, and changes in relationships with loved ones.

3. Follow-Up Care: After completing cancer treatment, survivors will need to continue with follow-up care, which may include regular check-ups, imaging tests, and blood work to monitor for any signs of recurrence.

4. Lifestyle Changes: To reduce the risk of cancer recurrence, survivors may need to make lifestyle changes such as adopting a healthy diet, exercising regularly, avoiding

tobacco and alcohol, and managing stress.

5. Support Networks: Many cancer survivors find that having a support network of family, friends, and other survivors can be helpful in adjusting to life after cancer.

It's important to note that life after cancer treatment can be challenging, but many survivors are able to resume their normal lives with some adjustments. It's also important for survivors to be kind to themselves and seek support if needed.

Chapter 6

Overcoming Fear and Anxiety

A. Techniques for emotional and mental wellness

Cancer can take a toll on a person's mental and emotional health. Coping with the diagnosis, treatment, and uncertainty can be overwhelming, and it is important to take steps to maintain mental and emotional

wellness. Below are a few
methods that could be beneficial;

1. Seek support: Join a
   cancer support group or
   talk to a therapist to get
   emotional support. It can
   be helpful to talk to others
   who are going through a
   similar experience.
2. Incorporating mindfulness:
   Incorporating mindfulness
   into your routine can aid in
   reducing stress and anxiety
   levels. You might consider
   practicing meditation,
   deep breathing, or yoga to
   achieve this.
3. Stay active: Exercise has
   been shown to improve
   mood and reduce stress.
   Talk to your doctor about
   safe exercise options.
4. Eat well: Eating a healthy
   diet can improve your
   mood and energy levels.
   Strive for a diet that
   includes a variety of fruits,
   vegetables, whole grains,
   and lean proteins.
5. Stay connected: Cancer
   can be isolating, but it is
   important to stay
   connected to friends and

family. Make time for social activities and stay in touch with loved ones.

6. Get enough sleep: Getting enough sleep is important for mental and emotional wellness. Try to establish a regular sleep schedule and create a relaxing bedtime routine.

7. Practice self-care: Take time for yourself each day to do something you enjoy, such as reading, listening to music, or taking a bath.

8. Manage stress: Stress can worsen mental and emotional health. Give a try on stress-reducing techniques such as deep breathing, meditation, or yoga.

Remember that taking care of your mental and emotional health is just as important as taking care of your physical health. If it's becoming an obstacle, reach out for help. Your healthcare team can provide resources and support.

B. Techniques to overcome the fear and anxiety

As a cancer patient, it is common to experience fear and anxiety. These emotions can be overwhelming and can make it difficult to cope with the diagnosis and treatment. However, there are steps you can take to help manage these feelings and improve your quality of life:

1. Seek support: It is important to have a support system to help you cope with your emotions. This can include family, friends, support groups, or a therapist.
2. Stay informed: Learning about your diagnosis, treatment options, and prognosis can help you feel more in control of your situation. Speak with your healthcare professionals and ask necessary questions.
3. Practice relaxation techniques: Activities like deep breathing, meditation, yoga, or

listening to calming music
can help you relax and
reduce anxiety.

4. Exercise regularly:
   Physical activity can help
   reduce stress and anxiety.
   Talk with your healthcare
   provider about what kind
   of exercise is safe for you
   to do during treatment.
5. Take care of yourself: It is
   important to take care of
   yourself physically and
   emotionally. Make time
   for things you enjoy and
   prioritize self-care.
6. Consider talking to a
   professional: A therapist
   or counselor can help you
   work through your fears
   and anxieties in a safe and
   supportive environment.

Remember, it is normal to feel
fear and anxiety as a cancer
patient. By taking steps to
manage these emotions, you can
improve your overall well-being
and feel more in control of your
situation.

Chapter 7

Treatment Options

A. Surgery

Surgery is one of the main treatment options for cancer, and it is often used to remove tumors that are localized and have not spread to other parts of the body. The goal of cancer surgery is to remove as much of the cancerous tissue as possible, while minimizing damage to healthy tissues and organs.

The specific type of surgery that is used for cancer treatment will depend on a number of factors, including the type and stage of the cancer, the size and location of the tumor, and the patient's overall health. Some common types of cancer surgery include:

1. Curative surgery: This type of surgery is used to remove the entire tumor, along with any nearby lymph nodes that may be affected by cancer. It is often used for early-stage cancers and can be highly effective in

preventing the cancer from spreading.

2. Palliative surgery: This type of surgery is used to relieve symptoms caused by cancer, such as pain or breathing difficulties. It is not intended to cure the cancer, but rather to improve the patient's quality of life.

3. Reconstructive surgery: This type of surgery is used to restore function or appearance to a body part that has been affected by cancer surgery. For example, breast reconstruction may be performed after a mastectomy.

In some cases, surgery may be used in combination with other cancer treatments, such as radiation therapy or chemotherapy. The specific treatment plan will depend on the individual patient and the type of cancer they have.

B. Chemotherapy

Chemotherapy is a type of cancer treatment that involves the use of drugs to destroy cancer cells. Chemotherapy drugs work by targeting rapidly dividing cells, which is a hallmark of cancer cells. However, these drugs can also affect normal cells in the body that divide rapidly, such as those in the bone marrow, hair follicles, and digestive tract, leading to side effects.

There are several chemotherapy options for cancer treatment, and the choice of drugs depends on the type of cancer, the stage of the disease, and the overall health of the patient. Here are some commonly used chemotherapy drugs and their uses:

1. Cyclophosphamide: Used to treat breast cancer, leukemia, lymphoma, and ovarian cancer.

2. Cisplatin: Used to treat bladder, lung, ovarian, and testicular cancer.

3. Doxorubicin: Used to treat breast cancer, leukemia, lymphoma, and lung cancer.

4. Fluorouracil: Used to treat breast cancer, colon cancer, and stomach cancer.

5. Paclitaxel: Used to treat breast cancer, ovarian cancer, and lung cancer.

6. Methotrexate: Used to treat leukemia, lymphoma, and breast cancer.

7. Vinblastine: Used to treat
lymphoma, testicular cancer, and
bladder cancer.
8. Vincristine: Used to treat
leukemia, lymphoma, and lung
cancer.
These drugs are usually given in
combination with other drugs,
and the treatment regimen varies
depending on the specific cancer
and the patient's response to the
treatment. Chemotherapy can be
administered orally,
intravenously, or topically,
depending on the drug and the
cancer being treated.

C. Radiation

Radiation therapy is frequently
used as a treatment for cancer. It
uses high-energy radiation to kill
cancer cells and shrink tumors.
There are several types of
radiation therapy which includes:
1. External beam radiation
therapy: External beam radiation
therapy is a form of radiation
treatment where high-energy
radiation is directed from a
machine outside the body
towards the cancerous area. It is
usually given on an outpatient
basis over several weeks.

2. Brachytherapy: In this type of radiation therapy, radioactive sources are placed inside the body near the cancer cells. This can be performed for a temporary or permanent reason.

3. Stereotactic radiosurgery (SRS) and stereotactic body radiation therapy (SBRT): These are specialized forms of radiation therapy that deliver high doses of radiation to small, well-defined tumors. They are often used to treat brain tumors or tumors in other parts of the body that are difficult to reach with traditional radiation therapy.

4. Proton therapy: This type of radiation therapy uses protons instead of X-rays to treat cancer. Proton therapy is often used for cancers that are close to critical organs or structures, such as the brain, spine, or prostate.

The type of radiation therapy that is best for a particular person depends on many factors, including the type and stage of the cancer, the location of the tumor, and the person's overall health. A radiation oncologist can help determine the most

appropriate type of radiation
therapy for a particular person.

Immunotherapy

Immunotherapy is a form of
cancer treatment that assists the
body's immune system in
targeting and destroying cancer
cells. It works by either
stimulating the immune system
to attack cancer cells or by
providing the immune system
with additional components to
enhance its ability to fight
cancer.
There are several types of
immunotherapy options for
cancer treatment, including:
1. Monoclonal antibodies: These
are lab-made antibodies that are
designed to attach to specific
proteins on the surface of cancer
cells. This can help the immune
system recognize and attack
cancer cells.
2. Immune checkpoint inhibitors:
These drugs block proteins on
cancer cells or immune cells that
can inhibit the immune system's
ability to recognize and attack
cancer cells.
3. CAR T-cell therapy: This is a
type of immunotherapy that

involves modifying a patient's T cells in a lab and then reinfusing them into the patient's body to recognize and attack cancer cells.

4. Cancer vaccines: These vaccines work by stimulating the immune system to recognize and attack cancer cells.

5. Cytokines: These are proteins that can help regulate the immune response and stimulate immune cells to attack cancer cells.

6. Adoptive cell transfer: This is a type of immunotherapy that involves removing immune cells from a patient, modifying them in a lab to recognize and attack cancer cells, and then reinfusing them into the patient's body.

The type of immunotherapy used will depend on the type and stage of cancer, as well as other individual patient factors. Immunotherapy has shown promising results in treating various types of cancer, but it's important to discuss with your doctor whether it's an appropriate option for you.

Conclusion

Resources for cancer patients

There are many resources available for cancer patients. Here are a few:

1. American Cancer Society: Provides information and support to cancer patients and their families, as well as resources for finding treatment, financial assistance, and support groups.

2. National Cancer Institute: Provides information about different types of cancer, treatments, clinical trials, and support services for patients and their families.

3. CancerCare: Offers free counseling, support groups, education, and financial assistance for cancer patients and their families.

4. Cancer Support Community: Provides support groups, educational programs, and wellness activities for cancer patients and their families.

5. Livestrong Foundation: Provides support services for cancer survivors, including financial assistance, emotional

support, and access to fitness and wellness programs.

6. Patient Advocate Foundation: Provides assistance with navigating the healthcare system, insurance coverage, and financial issues related to cancer treatment.

7. Cancer Hope Network: Offers one-on-one support from trained volunteers who have gone through cancer themselves.

8. Stupid Cancer: Provides resources and support specifically for young adults with cancer.

These are just a few of the many resources available to cancer patients. Your doctor or treatment center may also be able to provide additional resources and support.